Contents

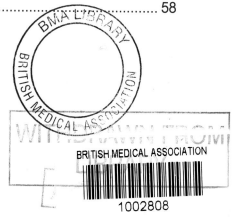

Prologue

MRCP PACES should be the final hurdle between you and the much coveted MRCP diploma.

It's at this stage in your career where you probably feel that your social and work lives are becoming blurred and consumed by PACES. You may also feel that the only thing between you and a consultant post is these nine letters.

If that sounds like you then I can hardly blame you. I remember feeling like this in 2015 right before I sat PACES but to be honest, life continues regardless of whether you pass or fail. A useful tip I learned to curb anxiety before a major life-event such as MRCP PACES or delivering an important presentation is to imagine your surroundings ten, twenty or even one hundred years from now when everyone including yourself will no longer be on the planet. The building you're currently in will still be here, occupied by different people and the events that happen today are very insignificant in the grand scheme of things. Practicing this type of **thought experiment** can be very humbling.

By the end of CT2, some of us can perform internal jugular vein cannulations and intercostals chest drains with relative ease but you'll soon realise that being a specialty registrar is a lot more than this.

During my time as a respiratory CT2, I remember having placed what must've been about twenty 12F chest drains into large malignant pleural effusions. However, as soon as I started ST3, I realised that the consultant had only let me do those particular drains "independently" because you couldn't exactly miss! Back then I could not even wield a proper thoracic ultrasound machine properly.

Now I'm looking forward to placing difficult 26Fr into empyemas, mastering bronchoscopy and competently manage complex outpatient respiratory cases. Even after (if) I achieve that I will still stare in awe when my consultants perform EBUS, thoracoscopy and indwelling pleural catheters with an air of aloofness in their demeanour.

Remember how happy you were when you passed finals? **MRCP PACES is simply another life event that all physicians have had to overcome at one point in their lives**. The next hurdle undoubtedly will be ensuring your CV looks good for ST3 applications.

By seeing MRCP PACES as only a checkpoint in your very long journey in becoming the best physician you can be, hopefully you'll understand that it's not the Mount Everest everyone makes it out to be. **Almost everyone eventually passes and goes on to become a consultant in their field**.

This guide will walk you through what you need to do to maximise your chances of **passing PACES on your first attempt and in just 8 weeks**.

Should you sit MRCP Part 2 or PACES first? Both simultaneously?!

"*Think back to a time when nursing staff approached you one after another with prescription charts, observation charts and fluid charts. Literally queuing up like customers at a lemonade stand. Your FY1 then runs into the room asking you about a gentleman who is vomiting bowlfuls of frank red blood. That's what attempting MRCP PACES and Part 2* **simultaneously** *feels like.*"

I overheard a consultant say that to one of the core medical trainees once and almost spat out my coffee in agreement!

It's not to say that attempting Part 2 and PACES is impossible but it's not the ideal situation to be in because your body and mind can only take so much abuse and stress at once. One of my fellow core medical trainees actually managed this feat in 2015 but it was out of necessity, rather than choice, otherwise she would've **delayed entry into a ST3 post**.

The reason why you should sit these exams separately is because they test different aspects of your clinical acumen. As a knowledge-intense exam, **Part 2 tests your memory and clinical application** of that knowledge over 9 hours in 2 days. I've been reliably informed that Part 2 is soon becoming a 6 hour exam over 1 day, just like Part 1. Lucky guys eh?

On the other hand, **PACES tests your ability to perform under pressure in real time** as well as **your communication skills and interaction with patients and relatives**. I would argue that those skills are equally, if not more important than knowledge in PACES.

The majority of you reading this guide will have already passed Part 2 and I congratulate you for having come so far but for those who are contemplating both together, think again because unless you absolutely have to then sit them separately. On the same note, I would definitely sit PACES after Part 2 as the knowledge you gain from the written exams will make PACES a lot easier. From my experience, the reverse isn't true.

Before We Start

"Work expands so as to fill the time available for its completion."

Parkinson's Law is the reason why 8 weeks should be enough time for PACES preparation. I'm sure there was a time in your life when you had many weeks or months to submit a piece of work for university. But somehow it was always the last week or even the last few hours or days before you started the project. Parkinson resonated so dearly with me during third year of medical school when we were assigned a piece of coursework with a deadline of two months. I ended up doing an all-nighter inside the university library the night before, cramming in 60 days of work in 10 hours!

I don't think I'm *that* unique in this regard. Need more evidence?

After passing MRCP Parts 1 and 2 Written in September and December 2014 I actually had 7 months until PACES in July 2015. Did I start revising ASAP? Of course, not.

I celebrated completion of the two exams with a holiday to Japan with my girlfriend. I then completely lost motivation and interest and began cruising auto-pilot through the remainder of my first core medical training year. And by cruising I don't mean I was very competent or that everything was achieved effortlessly. I just mean I went to work and returned home every day without showing enthusiasm to learn or do anything new. Surprisingly and unfortunately a lot of the juniors I work with nowadays give off this impression.

It wasn't until late-April 2015 before I began to panic and I subsequently joined a motivated study group. **It was during this eight week period I became quite serious and ended up passing MRCP PACES in early July 2015 on my first attempt**.

This guide documents the eight week period in my life when I took advantage of our friend Parkinson. This is the eight week technique I hope you can use to finally clear PACES so you can concentrate on more important things in your life, like spending time with your kids, or learning a registrar skill like endoscopy.

Before we start, we are going to carry out **two tasks**. The first is to find a **motivated study group or a partner** and the **second is to invest in a great course**.

Should you join a PACES group?

"You're the average of the five people you spend most time with."

This is one of my favourite quotes of all time because it's so simple yet so true. Success breeds success and a culture of failure breeds nothing but more failure and toxicity.

Apart from striving to become a better doctor every day, one of my other passions in life is becoming financially independent and I hope you can join me on that journey by visiting **www.UKdoctoronFIRE.com** where there are plenty of more MRCP tips and information on financial independence including quarterly passive income reports. Subscribing will give you access to my **exclusive monthly newsletters** that are unavailable to the general public.

The reason I digressed is that one of my greatest wishes is to find someone in real life to discuss passive income ideas. Unfortunately despite money being such an integral piece in our lives, it's still a relatively taboo topic so I'm struggling to find like-minded people.

How do I fully harness the power of that quote?

It's very simple actually – I surround myself with like-minded people in the mornings, during lunch and dinner and sometimes even before sleep. No, they're not imaginary friends but personal finance podcasts and blogs! With this technique, I have read and listened to hundreds of articles, podcasts and audiobooks on the topic to become the average of hundreds of successful people in this field.

You'll be glad to hear that MRCP PACES is far from being a taboo topic (unless that person has just failed) in your hospital and therefore you should have much more luck than me. To make your life easier, make it clear to everyone that you're trying to pass MRCP PACES and the word will spread naturally.

In addition to placing some pressure and accountability onto yourself, people are generally very helpful and will suggest going to a specific registrar or consultant who is very keen to teach. There may even be a PACES teaching program or whatsapp group if you're lucky.

If you can find a motivated partner or even better a motivated group then you should immediately offer to study together. **Avoid slackers** like the plague because even though they might be very nice people and great doctors you don't want to study with someone with no sense of urgency. Too much stress is annoying but some anxiety is necessary. You must avoid the additional stress of having to ensure your partner is coming to study!

Consultant and Registrar Teaching Rota

If you cannot find anyone to study with in your hospital, **now is the time to be proactive**. You have the option to listen to **PACES podcasts** which are freely available and created by like-minded people. Ask your local education department who will be able to point you in the right direction.

You also have the option to create your own PACES study group, with you as the first member. If you work in a relatively small hospital and you're the only trainee who's sitting the next PACES diet then you may have to invite or join a group from another hospital from the same trust. As long as you want MRCP badly enough, you'll find like-minded people and I can't stress enough how important it is to study with other people. With Parts 1 and 2, it's not a problem but for PACES you'll need to continuously critique each other's demeanour and communication skills throughout these eight weeks.

Something else to consider is a **consultant and registrar teaching rota**. Again, if this isn't available locally, be proactive and create one, or simply join one.

Ideally you want to create a "double sided rota" where on the first side; you have experienced consultants and senior registrars imparting their specialist wisdom. You'll understand when I say that some things simply cannot be learned from books and this is where their advice and discussions become critical.

The second side to your rota should contain CT2s and very junior registrars who have recently completed their MRCP PACES and can therefore teach you about the nuances of the exam. Imagine having someone who has just sat the exam at the same venue you'll be sitting PACES in.

PACES Triangle

Okay, now onto the good stuff.

PACES is difficult not because of the depth of knowledge required. In fact, due to **time restraints** and **choice of examiner**, you can only ever be asked on what a general physician should be expected to know about a given subject.

Firstly there are only 4 minutes for questions at stations 1 and 3 so playing your cards strategically shouldn't allow examiners more than 3 or 4 questions. Secondly, choice of examiner refers to the fact that the exam board would never ask a respiratory physician to examine you at the respiratory station nor would a gastroenterologist grill you about hepatitis. You'll most likely have two generalists at each station i.e. a cardiologist examining you at the renal station or an elderly physician examining you in the abdominal station.

Knowing the above, you should start your revision using what I call the **PACES Triangle**: knowledge, practice and presentation.

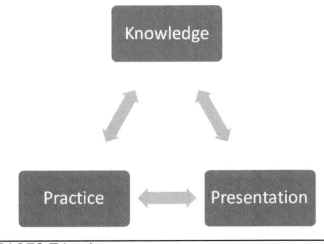

PACES Triangle

Knowledge, Practice & Presentation

"First comes knowledge."

First and foremost is **knowledge**.

Without knowledge you're unable to demonstrate your ability in the other aspects of the PACES triangle. You'll find that a significant amount of knowledge that you gained from the written exams will defend you against the examiners during question time. However, some knowledge won't be covered by Parts 1 and 2.

The books you should use for PACES knowledge are **both volumes of Clinical Medicine for the MRCP PACES by Mehta, Iqbal and Bowman**. They contain comprehensive descriptions of signs for most of the conditions you're likely to encounter in the exam and also have reasonable answers for the likely questions that you may be asked. I would highly recommend using this book for stations 1 and 3 for nothing else but to learn how to present signs to the examiners.

Whilst we're on the topic of answering the examiner's questions, I wanted to comment about **taking initiative**, or being proactive again. Consider the following exchange between examiner and candidate:

E: So you think the differential diagnosis is between pulmonary fibrosis and bronchiectasis. Why?

C: Due to presence of bilateral crepitations in both bases.

E: So how would you differentiate between them?

C: I would perform a CXR, spirometry and a CT chest.

E: And what would you expect to find?

When sitting any exam, knowledge is undoubtedly of paramount importance. **However, it never hurts us to think about the examiner**. Exceedingly few examiners like to ridicule candidates and on the same thread, most want us to do well and pass the exam with flying colours. Having recently organised the PACES exam at my local hospital as the organising registrar I can confirm that all the examiners wanted to pass candidates. **But they also wanted the day to pass a little quicker**.

If you were an examiner, the first few candidates might be a novelty, especially if the last time you examined was a few months or even a year ago. However by 11am, you're becoming a little hypoglycaemic and that morning coffee you had has long been used up. You cannot help but feel a little grumpy especially when you have to do all the work, and the candidate gives you one sentence answers.

Instead of making it tedious for the examiner, we can try this:

C: *After presentation of patient case* Therefore I feel that the differential diagnosis is between pulmonary fibrosis and bronchiectasis due to bibasal crepitations. I would try and differentiate between the two using spirometry which would demonstrate a restrictive ventilatory defect in pulmonary fibrosis but I would expect obstructive airflow in bronchiectasis. I would also request imaging in the form of CXR and CT scanning which may reveal tram track lines and the signet ring sign in bronchiectasis or honeycombing and ground glass changes in pulmonary fibrosis.

By extending your answer and ensuring it's of high quality, you'll use up time that would otherwise be occupied by potentially more difficult or **weird** questions that might deduct marks. I recently examined medical students during their end of year OSCEs and can vouch that I ran out of basic questions to ask for one particularly excellent student. Instead of the awkward silence, I then asked a more difficult question which would not be expected of her at that early stage.

More importantly you can actually steer the conversation in your preferred direction towards the knowledge you have revised. In the above example, you could easily continue the answer by talking about management of bronchiectasis and pulmonary fibrosis. Most examiners will be grateful (I was never stopped once) if you're producing a high quality answer and you're not simply rambling. I would even advocate extending your answers to 60 – 90 seconds long and never stopping during this time unless the examiners are visibly trying to get a word in.

"Practice makes perfect"

The second aspect of the PACES triangle is **practice**. You might be a good physician with a fountain of knowledge but the reality is that if you're unable to demonstrate this knowledge to the examiners, you'll perform poorly in MRCP PACES.

The first reason why lack of practice might fail you is when **you're unable to complete the examination stations in 6 minutes**. This is actually plenty of time to complete any one of the four major examinations and should still allow you some time to gather your thoughts before presentation and question time. You'll be at a significant disadvantage if you're not completing the examinations with time to spare.

Secondly with practice we become **slick**. Whilst examining 1st year medical students for their end-of-year OSCEs and during our examiner training, the clinical skills tutor warned us not to automatically pass students on all modalities just because they're excellent at one or two. Excellent of course encompasses being slick.

It's human nature to assume good looking people are smart, kind and rich but we don't actually have any evidence unless we get to know them. Similarly, if you're able to demonstrate slickness, examiners will automatically assume (fairly or otherwise) that you know what you're doing and that you're a great doctor. I'm sure those assumptions are true but I can't stress enough how many extra subconscious points you'll score with the examiners if you can demonstrate a gastrointestinal examination with ease because **first impressions matter**.

So how should you structure your practice?

When practising for MRCP PACES, it's imperative to remember that although recognising pathology is important, it's absolutely necessary to nail the **normal examination** first. It's slightly awkward performing five or six examinations on your PACES partner or a friendly colleague but if you have a partner then this shouldn't be a problem.

For the first couple of attempts, go through each and every step slowly to ensure you're ticking all the boxes. Next you can repeat this slightly quicker under timed conditions. I would encourage you to do at least ten normal examinations on each of stations 1 and 3 during the week you're studying that station. **Spread your "normal examination practice" throughout the eight weeks**. As you become more proficient and PACES draws closer, one or two examinations per week just to refresh your memory should suffice.

"Presentation, presentation, presentation"

If we think back to our driving tests, there was a theory exam prior to the practical. Similarly, we could technically navigate through the examination stations without properly understanding the significance of an ejection systolic murmur. **Presentation** is how you can demonstrate to the examiner that not only can you perform the movements, you also have the knowledge.

After passing both my written exams within the space of 3 months, my educational supervisor congratulated me. He was a very supportive consultant and gave me great advice that I write about in my other MRCP book. However, I remember one day he appeared particularly grumpy and casually mentioned out of nowhere that "*I think you might find PACES a bit difficult Rory*".

A similar thing happened with a fellow colleague. Despite being unable to clear Part 1, this colleague also directly said to me that I would struggle with PACES as it would be different from the written exams where only "hard work and study is required".

I didn't say anything in return to these comments but I knew why they made these comments.

I ended up passing MRCP PACES first time using the techniques I outline in this guide. My educational supervisor was very happy for me and proudly broadcasted it to the whole hospital. The colleague wasn't very convincing when he congratulated me.

Returning to the point I made about **first impressions**. I'm very quiet by nature so I'm someone who could be in a room full of people and not say a single word for the hour I'm there unless someone talks to me first. This is not because I'm cool, mean, or even disinterested. I genuinely find it difficult to shed my introverted personality but some people unfortunately mistake this for aloofness or even rudeness. In reality I just don't have anything to say. I am working on this.

Personally I think there are three different types of MRCP PACES candidates, depending on how you look at it. The first is essentially the one I've just described - naturally introverted and still so even in the work setting. The second type is the naturally extroverted individual but once in the work or exam setting, they freeze up and become introverts. Lastly is the naturally extroverted individual who can maintain this state regardless of the high pressure situation. Notice that for the purposes of this exam, the first two types are the same in the examiner's eyes.

Although humans like to categorise others, doing so doesn't really predict who'll pass MRCP PACES as I clearly demonstrated with my anecdote. If we're extroverts, I think it possibly increases our chances of passing but only if we don't ramble and go off in a tangent. If you're an introvert, this shouldn't hurt your chances because for those 2 hours and 5 minutes, you just need to become a **temporary extrovert**. As I described above, even if you're an introvert, you need to extend your answer as infinitely possible to demonstrate your knowledge and determination, and also take the pressure off the examiner to ask you the next undoubtedly harder question.

How did I pass MRCP PACES with relative ease? And how did I perform so well at the ST3 interview station where there was an interview station?

The secret really just is practice.

I'm definitely not someone who can just turn up at an event with no preparation and give a great speech or presentation. An easy way to find out whether you're gifted in this area is to imagine you've just examined a patient's cardiovascular system and you've found an irregularly irregular pulse and also a pansystolic murmur. Everything else was normal. Present to yourself in front of a mirror how you would present to an examiner under timed conditions.

If you're at the beginning of your revision you might not have given it much thought and just deliver the positive findings amongst some random negative findings. **Realise that even though you may present to your consultant or registrar every day on the ward rounds, the exam is entirely different and much more formal**.

Introverts may state that "Mr X is a middle aged man with an irregularly irregular pulse. On auscultation there was a pansystolic murmur. This is possibly in keeping with atrial fibrillation and mitral regurgitation" before running out of things to say. If you're a natural extrovert you may find yourself rambling more and not scoring points. You want to be in that **sweet spot** where everything you say adds value to your score sheet and you want to maintain this as long as possible.

The second point I wanted to touch upon was the topic of **colloquialisms** or **abbreviations**. After a few medical rotations as a FY2, CT1 and CT2, atrial fibrillation with a rapid ventricular response quickly gets shortened to "*fast AF*". An upper gastrointestinal bleed secondary to alcoholic liver disease and portal hypertension quickly becomes abbreviated to "*UGIB ALD*".

In the acute medical unit this is useful because it saves us time, but also demonstrates subconsciously to the listener on the phone that you're so experienced with dealing with this condition that you can call it fast AF. At this stage we would never dream of calling Langerhan's Cell Histiocytosis "*LCH*" even though some respiratory specialists do!

In the exam setting colloquialisms are very frowned upon so ensure that it's chronic obstructive pulmonary disease (not COPD) and myocardial infarction (not MI). Where possible, try and be as specific as you can and this goes back to the point of **extending everything**. This means clearly stating that it's a non-ST elevation myocardial infarction.

To shift your mindset in the lead up towards the exam, begin writing the full version of every condition in your clerk-ins in the acute medical unit. In the superficial exam setting, you will make yourself sound much more eloquent. Fast AF sounds very silly if you think about it and could actually mean fast as f***!

The last point I wanted to mention about presentation is to actually practice presenting. I would highly encourage you to invest in a **dictaphone** or a **voice recording application** on your smartphone. Do you hate the sound of your own voice? Me too. I think most of us do but there's no other solution to overcoming this.

For the above example of the irregularly irregular pulse and pansystolic murmur, start your preparation by imagining how you would present whilst you're on your commute or if you have a few minutes at work. Ideally you could present to a PACES partner but if it's your first attempt even that can be quite intimidating. When you're alone, present the case fully and as clearly as possible to the voice recorder and **replay it back to yourself**. **Critique yourself** and truly listen for stuttering or pertinent pieces of information being missed.

When you start off you may sound like this:

"I have just examined Mr X who is a...seventy um...something year old gentleman. He is comfortable at rest and is not in respiratory distress. On examination I found an irregularly irregular pulse at 84 beats per minute and a pansystolic murmur radiating to the axilla. This is probably mitral regurgitation associated with AF."

As you progress you'll soon sound like this:

"Mr X is an elderly gentleman who has kindly let me examine him. His main positive findings include an irregularly irregular pulse at 84 beats per minute and a pansystolic murmur radiating to the axilla. There was no clinical evidence of infective endocarditis, heart failure or anticoagulation. This is most likely mitral regurgitation associated with atrial fibrillation. Differentials of a pansystolic murmur can also include tricuspid regurgitation and ventricular septal defect and if I had time I would like to proceed to history taking and full respiratory examination. In terms of investigations, a 12 lead electrocardiogram would be useful to confirm atrial fibrillation. An echocardiogram would be important to characterise the valvular defect. If atrial fibrillation is confirmed then calculating the CHADSVASC score to stratify stroke risk would be my priority as this would guide anticoagulation therapy..."

Firstly, avoid trying to guess a patient's age. I've been in medicine for almost ten years now and I still frequently get it wrong. If the patient is young, call them young. If they're old, call them elderly. And if they're in between, call them middle aged. **Always be generous** though because you don't want to insult the examiner!

Secondly, every station has **important negatives**. In the above cardiology station it is important to mention the lack of clinical evidence of anticoagulation such as ecchymoses as you would expect patients with AF to be on anticoagulation.

Thirdly, always present your most likely diagnosis first. PACES cases are usually imperfect as it's not easy identifying "standard patients". In cases of mixed valvular disease, even the examiners have to rely on the echocardiogram report.

This is the reason why we follow up our most likely diagnosis with a differential. You should also continue (without pause) on **how you would differentiate between your differential diagnosis** because that is clearly the next question. If you were the examiner and the candidate gave three possible answers, you'd want them to narrow down the differential. Essentially, we are trying to predict their questions and make the process as easy as possible. I never did this for my preparation but you might want to consider writing down a candidate versus examiner interaction to hopefully place you in the shoes of the examiner. This may situate you in a better position to predict the next question.

Invest in a great course

"No-one fails after going to this course Rory"

Up until now I had never attended a course for any exam but MRCP PACES was admittedly a little different to any exam I had been to before. Everyone was raving about this London PACES course. I don't advertise other people's products (nor am I getting paid to do so) but in the interests of providing you with the best information I know about this topic, the course I attended was **PassPACES**. From memory I think the course organiser at the time was Rupa Bessant.

The exam costs about £700 but this course was double that. *Do I really need it?* The price of the four-day course was a whopping **£1,395** and in London that's the least of your worries. Accommodation, travel and subsistence brought that figure well over £2,000 or one month's salary.

I deliberated and deliberated some more before deciding I couldn't afford it and applied for the local hospital's PACES course instead. After all, it would cost one month's salary and I had rent and food still to pay for.

A few weeks before the local PACES course was due to start, it was cancelled due to insufficient delegate numbers and I immediately seized the opportunity to request for the trust to pay for this London PACES course.

Although I still ended up paying over £500 for accommodation and food, I'm grateful my trust paid for this course. The lesson from this story is *if you don't ask you don't get*. We should always request study leave allowance first before paying for courses ourselves because each trust receives money from their national education department to invest in us.

If your hospital hosts their own PACES course then it'll be difficult to justify them spending so much money but keep your eyes peeled for any opportunities that may arise.

The four-day course was very intense and spanned most of each day between 8am and 5pm. There were numerous patients with a wide range of pathology available for getting practical experience on. I actually took quite unwell after day 1 but because so much money was involved, I powered on for the remaining three days.

The organiser was very strict and the environment was so stressful that one of the candidates disappeared after day 2. For the days he was present he was very nervous and struggled during presentations. Personally I loved every minute of it because I felt like I was training for something really important, almost like in some type of boot camp. In reality, it's quite hard to justify spending £2,000 on top of the PACES fee.

Over the four days I saw a multitude of pathology and in fact one of the cases (**simultaneous pancreatic**

and kidney transplant) actually appeared in the exam. Having never done a renal SHO job before, I had never encountered this presentation until then so I'm really glad I attended the course.

You don't have to attend that specific course obviously but I've still yet to come across someone who bravely skips a PACES course before their exam. There are shorter two-day courses available for half the price so that's an alternative option but I'll let you do your own research on this one.

Weeks 1 and 2

Hopefully by now you have an idea of what it takes to pass MRCP PACES. In addition to having sound knowledge, you'll also need to demonstrate good organisational skills by structuring your preparation in 8 weeks around your busy CMT jobs.

We discussed the need to revise using a good PACES book to gain PACES-specific knowledge rapidly. We talked about practising examination skills and ultimately presentation skills using some form of voice recording tool.

Now we should think about how you should structure your eight weeks.

In **week 1**, I would advise working on your PACES triangle with regards to **Station 1: respiratory and abdominal**.

Week 2 should be focussed on **Station 3: cardiology and neurology**.

Monday – Respiratory
Tuesday – Respiratory
Wednesday – Respiratory
Thursday – Abdominal
Friday – Abdominal
Saturday – Abdominal
Sunday – Respiratory & Abdominal

Your first week should look something like the above. The reason I haven't specified whether you should be studying knowledge, practice or presentation is because there is no ideal way. Remember the study variation technique I taught in **MRCP Parts 1 and 2 Written Guide**? The way I studied for PACES was again using study variation. Studying for 3 or 4 hours from a textbook can get soul destroying very quickly. Instead, every day should be used to study knowledge, practice and presentation intermittently and so you may wish to spend an hour on each aspect per day for example.

Before you dive into respiratory, for example, you should decide the main conditions you're planning to revise. For instance, it would be prudent to include pulmonary fibrosis, collapse, pleural effusion, pneumonectomy and lobectomy, bronchiectasis, COPD and raised hemidiaphragm in your preparation. Therefore your revision may look like this:

Monday - Knowledge for pulmonary fibrosis, collapse and pleural effusion, practice respiratory examination for 20 minutes, presenting respiratory cases for 40 minutes
Tuesday - Knowledge for pneumonectomy and lobectomy, bronchiectasis, practice respiratory examination for 15 minutes, presenting respiratory cases for 40 mins
Wednesday - Knowledge for COPD and raise hemidiaphragm, practice respiratory examination for 10 mins, presenting respiratory cases for 40 mins

Sunday - skim through notes, do one full respiratory examination in 6 mins, present a few difficult cases

Remember not to excuse yourself from practising a full respiratory examination just because you're not in the hospital or there happens to be no patients with that particular sign on that day. A normal respiratory examination under timed conditions is just as good. At this stage, I'm sure we're all able to imagine what reduced breath sounds and a scar sounds and looks like. That's essentially what you'll find in a pneumonectomy or lobectomy. Being able to perform the examination with slickness and within 6 minutes is so much more important.

Stations 1 & 3
Comprehensive and correct physical examination technique
Detect physical signs
Construct differential diagnosis
Suggest sensible and appropriate investigation and management plans
Treat patient with dignity and respect

Main Objectives: Stations 1 & 3

Anxious candidates may look at this study plan and feel that it's careless or even slightly short. It's at this point that I would refer you back to Parkinson's Law. It's so much more important to have an overview of your preparation and be able to see the end of the tunnel. It's theoretically possible to study for tuberculosis, silicosis, sarcoidosis, all subsets of interstitial lung disease etc but the idea of MRCP PACES is to create a general physician who is competent in basic respiratory or basic gastroenterology.

Start off by spending 3.5 days studying respiratory, abdominal, cardiology and neurology each and ensure that you move onto the next phase of revision even if you don't feel 100% ready. You'll have time at the end of the eight weeks to revisit areas that you feel are lacking.

To end this chapter, the above table highlights the main aspects you'll be tested on in stations 1 and 3.

Week 3

"Medicine is 90% history and 10% examination"

I can't remember who said this to me but it really has a lot of truth in it. In reality it's more like 60% history, 35% investigations and less than 5% examination so I'm not sure what the PACES board are thinking when they allocate so few marks to history taking. Anyway, it is what it is.

This week should be spent honing your history taking skills. I'm not sure about you but at that stage there were a few things that I found quite embarrassing to ask about. I know I should've got rid of it after medical school but for some reason I managed to avoid taking a sexual health history on people presenting with chest pains and breathlessness on the acute medical unit!

In addition to being able to ask **key differentiating questions** you'll also be required to ask "awkward" questions with slickness. If you're really struggling to phrase things well on the spot, simply be truthful to the patient or actor. "*Apologies for asking this question but it's very relevant to your symptoms...*"

An example of a key differentiating question would be asking about a patient's occupation when they present with obstructive sleep apnoea. Station 2 History Taking is generally thought of as the easiest station because although a lot us may perform a quick 30 second examination of the chest, most of us will spend a good 10 minutes talking to our patients at the very least. By sheer time spent on history taking versus examination, **we should already be excellent at history taking**.

For me personally, history taking was the easiest station. Since PACES I don't remember ever performing a full respiratory examination on a patient. Tracheal deviation simply isn't a very practical sign because even when we find it, we would probably wait for the CXR before inserting an intercostal chest drain! In contrast, we would never dream of missing out anything from the history such as travel or smoking history or even their pets in a respiratory history taking station.

The main point is to differentiate yourself from a medical student taking a history. Anyone can take a good chest pain history using the SOCRATES acronym but in PACES they're testing whether you can create a reasonable differential diagnosis following your history. They also want to know whether you're able to stratify this chest pain into low, medium or high risk. What implications does this have? Does the patient need admitting or can they have outpatient investigations? Whilst SOCRATES is useful in a headache history, you'll also want to know if there are any features of increased intracranial pressure. Every history taking station has its own set of differentiating questions so remember it's not simply a tick box exercise of asking about their family history, smoking, alcohol and social history.

You have 14 minutes in the station for the entire history and it's generally one in which most candidates have some time to spare. The best strategy is to ask questions slowly but also simultaneously ask yourself what condition this could be. What are the differentials? What is the key issue the examiners are wanting me to address?

Throughout week 3 you should also practice each of the four major clinical examinations: respiratory, neurology, cardiology and abdominal **twice** just to maintain your slickness.

Station 2
Gather data from patient
Construct a differential diagnosis
Deal with concerns the patient may have
Construct a management plan that is explained to the patient clearly
Treat patient with dignity and respect

Main Objectives: Station 2

The above table documents the main areas examiners are assessing you in during your history taking encounter.

*I also wanted to mention that the **MRCP (UK) website currently contains 15 sample scenarios** specific to Station 2 that you might find very useful.*

Creating systematic presentations

Knowledge, Practice and Presentation are your three main pillars for MRCP PACES success.

By now hopefully you've either invested in a voice recording device or downloaded an equivalent application on your phone. You will have had time to practice in front of the mirror and unless you're naturally good at presenting patients in a systematic manner, hopefully you'll realise there's a lot of work to be done!

The reason why you want to create systematic presentations at this point in your revision is because now you have an overall idea of what the exam is about. You have also had a chance to revise history taking and examination for the major four systems and hopefully have had a look at some of the minor ones.

For example, when presenting in a **renal** station, you want to ask yourself a pre-determined set of questions and this goes for all the history taking and examination stations. Here's an example of your thought process:

1. What is the aetiology? The main causes of renal failure are hypertension and diabetes but you'll need to remember vasculitides and polycystic kidney disease and a couple of rare

ones. When examining, state you would like to check the BP and state you would like to perform a finger prick test or simply look for them on the patient's fingers! When history taking, do not just ask for a general family history, ask specifically for autosomal dominant polycystic kidney disease!

2. Current RRT?
3. Previous RRT? The renal physicians are going to slap me for saying this but the good news is that they won't be examining you in the renal station. There are only three forms of renal replacement therapy: renal transplant, haemodialysis (via fistulae or central venous catheter) and peritoneal dialysis. It goes without saying to look for scars in the abdomen, the neck and anterior chest and the abdomen. Oh, and feel for a mass under a scar.
4. Mention that the RRT is functioning well (or not). Only stable patients are used for PACES examinations and therefore 99/100 times you'll only need to mention that the RRT is working. Obviously if a patient is uraemic and confused you don't say that.
5. Any complications? This is where it can get slightly confusing. Essentially you want to think about what medications such a patient would be taking. Steroids, ciclosporin and tacrolimus are probably the most common ones but be aware of the other ones. Not only can finger prick marks alert you to the aetiology of end stage renal failure, bear in mind that these immunosuppressants can

lead to diabetes. This is an area where you can potentially impress the examiners.

The reason why I've specifically mentioned the renal station is because although we've performed the neurology or abdominal examinations many times before, we were never taught the "renal examination" or at least I never was.

Bringing all this together, your presentation would go along the lines of this: "Mr X is a middle aged gentleman I have just examined presenting with **whatever symptoms the scenario states**. This gentleman most likely has end stage renal failure with a renal transplant. The aetiology is most likely diabetes mellitus due to the presence of fingertip prick marks but differential diagnoses would include hypertension and vasculitis. His current renal replacement therapy is a functioning right renal transplant as evidenced by a right iliac fossa scar with an underlying smooth and firm mass dull to percussion. The presence of a brachiocephalic fistula in his left arm suggests previous haemodialysis. There are no other scars on the anterior chest wall, neck or abdomen to suggest other forms of renal replacement therapy. The renal transplant appears to be functioning well due to Mr X's euvolaemic state and absence of confusion and asterixis. The presence of gum hypertrophy may also suggest that this gentleman is taking an immunosuppressant such as ciclosporin. To complete my assessment I would like to take a full history and perform bedside investigations such as a urinalysis to look for microscopic haematuria, proteinuria and glucose. I would also check blood tests including FBC, U&Es, HbA1c....and renal tract ultrasound..."

I'm sure you get the idea now but don't let your presentation stop. There are actually so many more things you could steer the conversation to. The only exceptions to this rule are during an unexpected emergency or if the examiner looks like they're trying to get a word or a question in!

Oh, and remember end stage renal failure is not a diagnosis – you'll be expected to come up with a cause!

Weeks 4, 5 and 6 - Station 5

In weeks 4, 5 and 6 you should start preparing for station 5. If you examine the marking scheme station 5 is worth a third of the marks of the entire exam and as such your time allocation should reflect this. If you have 8 weeks to study for PACES you should dedicate around 3 weeks to this station alone.

The best resources I would recommend for station 5 are the **PACES course**, **videos** and the textbook **An Aid to the MRCP PACES by Ryder Station 5 Volume 3**.

Station 5 consists of two 10-minute short clinical encounters attempting to decipher how you would interact with a patient in real life. Time is truly the limiting factor and is definitely the difference between passing and failing. Therefore every question and examination should be focused and purposeful. Your systemic enquiry should literally be one question.

The other difficulty with station 5 is how to practice and present cases. It's reasonably straightforward to create systems when presenting a station 1 or 3 case as I demonstrated above. There's a clear linear thought process that you can demonstrate to the examiner to confirm your knowledge, practice and presentation skills. How can we do that with an awkward station 5 case?

This is where I think the **Ryder textbook is a life-saver for station 5**, and this was how I used his book.

The book begins with an examination routine section where it teaches you a systematic way of examining seemingly random but very relevant **mini-systems** including pulses, fundi, hands and even skin. Why is that useful? Most core medical trainees probably haven't had the opportunity to attend very many dermatology or ophthalmology clinics and therefore having a simple routine to examine skin or the eyes is invaluable.

After you learn the system, the PACES triangle states you should now practice doing this. Practice the thyroid examination so much that reaching for that tendon hammer is second nature. This means performing this examination several occasions initially on your partner and maintaining this slickness throughout your eight weeks.

And once you're comfortable with performing the examination, you should start working on the last corner of the triangle: presentation.

A resource is only as good as the student, just like a tool is only as good as the handyman. You can read the Ryder textbook passively and find the examination findings and their example presentation of dermatomyositis interesting. But if you don't practice that "dermatomyositis examination" and you don't know how to present such a case, you're not actively increasing your chances of passing PACES.

Practice a hypothyroidism or a dermatomyositis presentation to your voice recorder.

Always remember that PACES revision should be **30% input and 70% output**. 30% of the time can be spent reading textbooks and watching videos – these are passive actions or input. The other remaining 70% should be used effectively to produce movement and voice; movement in the form of practising the examination skills and voice in the form of vocalising your presentation.

Initially you may open the book and be overwhelmed by the sheer number of cases but one piece of good news is that you only need to learn one examination routine for each mini-system. Regardless of whether the patient has retinitis pigmentosa or diabetic retinopathy, your ophthalmology examination will always be the same.

On the topic of examination practice, try not to make excuses for yourself. If you don't have an ophthalmoscope that evening, use a pen and practice all the other movements on your partner, making sure you use your right eye to examine their right eye and so on. Then when you do have access to an ophthalmoscope, you can concentrate on how to adjust its settings and switch it on.

The final thing I wanted to mention about Ryder was that after reading the initial patient clinical encounter blurb, I would hide the author's presentation and answers. I would read the examination findings once and try to present the case to myself out loud. My initial attempts were always cringe worthy but I would uncover the author's standard presentation afterwards and compare their written response to my verbal one. I would then rinse and repeat after a few minutes. Before very long, the key phrases were "second nature". Not only did I have knowledge, I could also demonstrate it through my rehearsed presentation skills.

In addition to a PACES course and Ryder's book, I would recommend using a PACES website. Outputting is much more difficult than absorbing information i.e. inputting because the latter requires a lot less effort. Outputting is also difficult because you're producing work that's at the mercy of others' judgement. But outputting is where you become a real PACES candidate.

When you're exhausted from all the reading, practising and presenting, you have the option to open a video and watch one of your predecessors perform the examination under standard and timed conditions. The website with the best videos is probably **Pastest** in my experience, and again I'm not paid to say so.

One advantage of watching other people is that you can incorporate their good habits into your routine whilst ensuring you oust their bad ones.

Weeks 7 and 8

The timetable for your final two weeks will be very dependent on how your revision has gone so far. **For each of the first six weeks, regardless of whether you're ready or not, I would strongly urge you to continue to the next stage of revision**. Reason being we'll never feel ready because medicine is just such a vast topic. Even still hopefully you've managed to cover all of the major and common stations. The last two weeks will be to clean up anything you feel you've missed or are worried about.

Note that common in PACES does not mean common in real life. An example of this would be acromegaly which comes up relatively frequently in the exam but hardly ever in hospital.

I would spend a few days during this fortnight on station 4: communication skills. But for the majority of current practising doctors, this should be a relatively simple station. The station 4 I had was counselling a woman on her father who was slowly dying from the complications associated with Parkinson's disease. Whilst it requires you to have some knowledge of the condition, most of the scenario revolves around your ability to elicit the daughter's **ideas, concerns and expectations (ICE)** and even a lay person can score highly in those areas.

Station 4
Guide and organise the interview with the subject
Explain clinical information
Apply clinical knowledge, including ethics, to management of case or situation
Provide emotional support
Treat the patient with dignity and respect

Main Objectives: Station 4

It goes without saying that communication skills is much more than this so you'll need to brush up on **how to deliver bad news** and **reinforce your knowledge on basic concepts like the mental health act, confidentiality and the four bioethical principles and more**.

Otherwise your last two weeks should be spent plugging any perceived holes you may have in your knowledge, practice and presentation. If differentiating between an ejection systolic and pansystolic murmur is difficult, now is the time to seek the help of a friendly cardiologist. If skin doesn't make any sense, then it's time to open the Ryder book and start focusing on that chapter first. The next day you should visit the dermatology ward or clinic for some practice.

Be honest. If presentation is troubling you, spend the next week literally presenting one hundred cases! It's not rocket science.

*I also wanted to mention that the **MRCP (UK) website currently contains 23 sample scenarios** specific to Station 4 that you might find very useful.*

MRCP PACES Marking Scheme

They say that knowing the marking scheme is half the battle, and having past papers is probably the second half.

At the beginning of the exam you'll be given 16 marksheets with verbal instructions to write your name and candidate number on each. Although there are only 5 stations, there are actually 8 separate scenarios (see table) and two examiners at each scenario, totalling 16.

Station	Scenario	Examiners
1	Respiratory	A + B
1	Abdominal	A + B
2	History Taking	C + D
3	Neurology	E + F
3	Cardiology	E + F
4	Communication Skills	G + H
5	Brief Clinical Encounter 1	I + J
5	Brief Clinical Encounter 2	I + J

MRCP PACES: Eight Scenarios

Seven separate skills are assessed in the MRCP PACES examination and each scenario tests a different combination of these skills. In reality, the marks are extremely binary and can be summarised as follows. If the examiner feels you're unsatisfactory in a particular skill, you're given a 0; borderline and you're given a 1 and if you're satisfactory then you're awarded a 2. Note that you just have to be satisfactory, whatever that means, and that there are no extra points for being excellent.

The second table details the seven skills that you'll be assessed on:

	Skills	Pass Mark
A	Physical Examination	16/24
B	Identifying Physical Signs	14/24
C	Clinical Communication	11/16
D	Differential Diagnosis	17/28
E	Clinical Judgement	19/32
F	Managing Patient Concerns	10/16
G	Maintaining Patient Welfare	28/32
	Total Pass Mark	**130/172**

MRCP PACES Pass Marks

To pass MRCP PACES, you'll need to score 130 out of the available 172 AND pass each separate skill. Additionally, if you score exactly 28/32 in patient welfare, the examiners will assess your performance and decide whether you pass or not, regardless of your total test score.

	Clinical Skill	Skill Descriptor
A	Examination	Correct, thorough, systematic, fluent and professional technique
B	Identifying Signs	Correctly; don't make up signs
C	Communication	Elicit relevant, systematic, thorough, fluent and professional history. Explain info similarly.
D	Differential	Sensible
E	Judgement	Select or negotiate sensible management plans. Select appropriate investigations and treatment. Apply clinical knowledge and ethics.
F	Managing Concerns	Seek, detect, acknowledge and address concerns. Listen and demonstrate empathy.
G	Maintaining Welfare	Respect, comfort, safety and dignity.

From this information, we can conclude two points.

As you can see from the fourth table, **station 5** assesses you on all 7 skills and therefore is worth 56 marks out of the available 172, or essentially **one third of the exam**. It is of utmost important you dedicate two to three full weeks towards station 5 as we discussed.

Station	Encounter	Skills Assessed
1	Respiratory	A B D E G
1	Abdomen	A B D E G
2	History	C D E F G
3	Cardiovascular	A B D E G
3	Neurology	A B D E G
4	Communication	C E F G
5	Station 5 (1)	ABCDEFG
5	Station 5 (2)	ABCDEFG

MRCP PACES: Skills Assessed in each "Station"

Secondly, **skill "G" or managing patient welfare is so crucial to your overall success in the exam**. Together with skill "E", clinical judgement, it's assessed in all eight clinical scenarios and by definition contains most of the marks. In fact, together they comprise 64 of your total 172 marks.

As the third table suggests, **managing patient welfare is simply actions we would take as a human being**, let alone as a doctor. There is no reason why you can't respect another human being whilst keeping them dignified, comfortable and safe.

Read the scenario. Then read the scenario again.

There have been two occasions in my life where I have examined candidates in a clinical exam.

The first time was during a PACES course and mock exam that I somehow managed to become an examiner in during CT1, right after I passed the exam in 2015. I remember sitting next to a ST6 registrar and we were both examining candidates during the mock PACES. We then took turns grilling them and giving them on the spot feedback which did feel uncomfortable as I was still so junior.

The second time was very recently when I helped examine medical students in their OSCEs.

The main thing that struck me for both encounters was the number of candidates who failed to **read the question properly**. And what happens when we mis-read a question or don't read it at all? Even if we've properly prepared we end up looking like we're struggling and it gives off a terrible first impression.

Many scenarios are quite lengthy but you can normally take the question sheet into the station and refer back to it anytime. Also, nothing is preventing you from apologising to the patient and referring back to the question because nobody can expect you to remember all the clinical details like BP, cholesterol level and how many cats and dogs the patient has.

Something to be aware of is a question that has multiple bullet points or stems. For example, a communication station such as the Parkinson's disease one may ask you to:

- Explain the situation to the daughter
- Propose any treatments
- Advise on prognosis

In a question like this, you will need to prioritise these three bullet points to maximise your marks. Failing to address one of them is like automatically surrendering a third of your marks for that station. Insane.

Non-technical skills

Nobody pays much attention to **non-technical skills** anymore and out of everyone I know, medics are the most pragmatic of people. As I mentioned in my first MRCP book, a significant portion of candidates spent the time prior to the written exams and during their lunch breaks reading from textbooks and performing practice questions. However I firmly believe in resting your mind and letting yourself recover during these much needed rest periods.

I'm ashamed to admit this but recently I failed my advanced life support (ALS) re-certification course. I talk about it in quite a lot of detail on my blog **www.UKdoctoronFIRE.com** but essentially what happened was that I underestimated the exam and also neglected the non-technical skills.

My mind had become very foggy from weeks and months of poor dieting and poor sleep, to the point where I struggled to focus, let alone write these sentences. It seemed to just creep up on me and was not a simple act of neglect. I had worked out intensely, lifting heavy weights (squatting 90kg+ and benching 80kg+ for repetitions with good form) three times per week and ate a lot of chicken so I wasn't being completely neglectful but it just wasn't enough. I was becoming mentally slow and physically lethargic and the reason was because I was eating too much junk food.

I also naively scheduled my ALS exam at the end of a twelve day work fortnight and was absolutely exhausted when I got to the friday evening exam time. I think I'm invincible at 27 but clearly I need to sort my life out.

The solution I found is to **be honest with yourself**. Compared to a time in your life when your mind was very sharp, how do you fare now? If you're only functioning at 70% how can you get closer to your maximum potential?

If your mind is foggy or you're feeling lethargic, then set aside some time before or after work to **exercise**. Some candidates immediately protest that there isn't enough time during these eight weeks to study but I would rather sacrifice one hour, three times per week to exercise than to study because it's just that important. Not only does exercise combat feelings of anxiety and depression, it also makes you much more resistant to illness. Comfort food is of course mandatory and please don't think for a moment I only eat chicken and broccoli. However try to always have two meals in the day where you have some **protein and greens**. And try and cut out all drinks that aren't **water or coffee/tea**.

Research your PACES centre to see what their "specialty" is, because every hospital has a specialty. Even if you "only" live one hour away from the hospital, it's worth paying for a hotel and staying close by the night before. Don't underestimate what the effect of being stuck in traffic for one hour will have on your feelings and performance. Make sure everything is accounted for including your dinner, the breakfast before the exam and your parking space. Will there be taxis on Monday at 830am? Regardless of what you read or hear, just wear what you wear to work. Don't make me regret writing that last sentence guys!

PACES Fast Track

Not many candidates know about this **PACES "secret"** even though it's on the MRCP website. To be fair, it does spontaneously disappear from time to time, and yes I'm that sad I still check it from time to time. If you're a CT2 applying or in the process of applying for a ST3 post then you're in for a treat.

Life has no guarantee and even the best prepared candidates can have a bad or unlucky day. The people who have created this exam recognise this and essentially give the candidates a **SECOND TRY IN THE SAME SITTING**.

To be eligible, you either have to be a **current CT2 working in the UK** as we've just mentioned, or **you have to prove that you're applying for a ST3 post at the next round**.

Due to limited capacity they also have a prioritisation process where they'll preferentially accept applications from current CT2s working in UK, followed by those who are not but are applying for ST3 in the next round with two or fewer previous attempts at PACES. Last in line are those who are in the same latter situation with more than two previous attempts.

The way I understand how it works is that say you are a CT2 approaching August changeover and still have PACES to overcome. You can pay for two PACES exams in the same sitting. If you fail the first, touchwood, then you get a second opportunity to pass so that your failure hopefully doesn't delay your entry to ST3. This is a frustrating barrier that prevented a good colleague of mine becoming a haematology registrar recently.

If you pass first time, they simply refund your money for the second exam so it's a win-win solution. Make sure you apply early and don't miss out on this opportunity that so many people overlook.

Failing PACES

"If you fall seven times, you just have to get up eight times."

"Doing the same thing over and over again expecting different results is the definition of insanity."

If you fail despite your best efforts then I refer you to the above quotes.

Everyone makes mistakes and that's why pencils come with erasers. I even failed a simple exam like ALS and I thought it was impossible to fail! But I reflected on the things I could change and I took **responsibility**.

I cannot stress this enough but you must **request detailed feedback** from the examiners immediately. Whilst you're waiting for their reply, take a few days off everything to **reflect** on anything you could have improved upon.

I don't want to bull**** you or sugarcoat anything but be harsh about yourself. If you're terrible at recognising murmurs then spend all your clinic time in the cardiology department prior to your next sitting. If English isn't your first language and you think that played a major part of your downfall then from now until your next exam, speak nothing but English even if it's outside your comfort zone.

Be really really harsh. If you need a haircut get one. If you're overweight, lose some weight. Even if you can't think of anything you did wrong, **it was probably still your fault**. Wear a different shirt and buy a new pair of shoes just so you're in the mindset that you need to change.

The most dangerous thing you can do after failing an exam is feeling like you're already the best you can be. I've seen candidates who have great medical knowledge but very poor communication skills failing three times in a row. They don't ask for any advice and still feel like nothing needs to be changed.

If you have any questions or comments, please don't hesitate to contact me via rory@ukdoctoronfire.com. I look forward to hearing from you. Good luck!

Printed in Great Britain
by Amazon